Contents

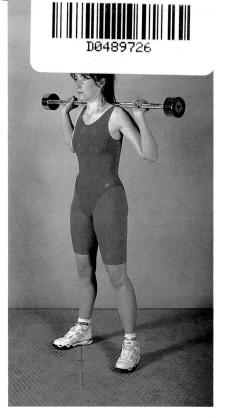

Acknowledgements
Text by John Lear, Director of Coaching
British Weight Lifters'
Association.
The publishers would like to thank Puma
UK Limited for their contribution to this
book.

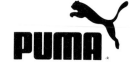

Thanks to Joanne Cripps and Peter May for
demonstrating the exercises.
Thanks also to the staff at Bisham Abbey
for use of the facilities there.
Front cover photograph by Grant Pritchard.
All other photographs by Nigel Farrow.

Note Throughout the book weight
trainers are referred to individually as
'he'. This should, of course, be taken
to mean 'he or she' where appropriate.

Introduction

It is often believed that people who are
strong are not necessarily fit, and that
the use of weights will not produce systematic fitness but muscular strength
only. To some degree this can be so,
depending on the methods of training
that are employed. For instance, by lifting very heavy weights for low repetitions great strength can be developed;
but the effects on the heart, circulation
and breathing systems will be minimal.
At the other end of the scale, lifting
very light weights for very high repetitions may well affect the cardio-
vascular and circulo-respiratory systems; the effect on building strength
and power will be low. Since fitness,
which can be both general and specifically related to sport, is made up of
stamina, strength, flexibility and speed,
weight training can play a most important part in achieving these essential
aspects of the whole development.

*Know The Game Fitness Training with
Weights* deals with the overload principle both for general and specific pur-
poses. It outlines progressive methods
of training and gives clear descriptions
of the basic exercises.

I hope that this form of exercise will
give you great pleasure in performance
and measurable achievement.

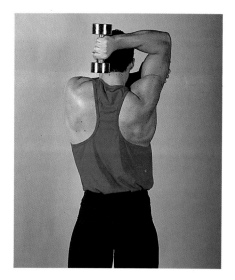

Fitness considerations

The principal objective of following any exercise programme is to develop and improve fitness. Often only a vague idea of what this means is understood and is related to a hope for a better sense of well being, a limitation of the chances of becoming ill, reduced body weight, and so on. If one asks the question, 'Why do you wish to become fitter?', answers such as 'If I am fitter I shall be able to conduct my life more effectively', 'I shall have a more attractive and acceptable physical appearance' or 'Fitness is an insurance for my health as I get older', are typical. A young person may view training from the point of view that 'I shall be able to play my sport with greater success.' All these statements are realistic and valid and lead to a definition of fitness as *the improved ability to adapt successfully to the stress, both physical and mental, of an individual's lifestyle.*

Our lifestyles are affected by our environment, both economically and socially, our family, our attitude to health and work, and our personal ambitions. These areas often place stress on us mentally, but it is through physical activity that our lives may be modified – especially by recognising that the body is the one machine that improves its functions by progressive loading. Exercise programmes and styles, when controlled by a progressive method, are essential to improved physical and mental performance and protection.

Components of fitness

Cardio-vascular and circulo-respiratory (stamina) fitness

This is the ability of the heart, lungs and circulatory systems to provide the muscles with nutrients and oxygen and to remove waste products during sustained physical activity. The working of the heart must be very efficient in order that fitness, particularly for sport, can be achieved. We need to develop these organs of circulation and respiration in order to improve our speed of recovery. Of course, this will allow the athlete to train harder, to recover more quickly from bouts of activity, and where appropriate to perform better under the challenge of competition. Since the heart is a muscle, training will improve its function. The benefit of this is an increase in *stroke* volume, i.e. the amount of blood pumped per beat.

Muscular endurance

This is the ability of a muscle or muscle group to work for very long periods of time without getting fatigued. Many sports involve this type of activity which may last for hours or days. Often, however, since these activities are competitive, the ability to produce power for certain periods within the overall timescale is essential.

Strength

This is the maximum force a muscle or muscle group can generate against a given resistance. Strength is often seen as a 'raw' quality. An extreme example is *dinamometric* application, where the participant exerts maximum effort against immovable objects or weights. This is known as 'isometric' work (*see* page 7).

Power

Power is the relationship between strength and speed. Most power events and displays are of a comparatively short duration. Power production also relates very closely to the particular skill or skills involved in an activity. It can be said to be the most important quality in any successful sporting performance, and in combination with endurance produces the highest levels of physical achievement.

Flexibility

In all skill performance, a full range of movement is essential. The ability to move limbs at the joints easily through their full and natural range of movement is necessary in both sport and in life. Flexibility is easily lost. Remember that all weight training exercises must be performed through the complete range of the exercise movement. Flexibility is best achieved by non-ballistic methods.

In the development of all of the above components of fitness, weight training can play a very important role. It is a controlled form of exercise that can be performed with free weights or weight machines to 'overload' the systems, especially the muscular system (*see* page 12).

The potential benefits of weight training can be listed as follows:

- increase in strength
- increase in speed
- increase in muscular endurance, leading to . . .
- increase in stamina
- increase in flexibility and full mobility
- increase in strength around joints, preventing injury
- rapid rehabilitation of muscles following injury
- potential decrease in body fat
- consequent improvement in shape and appearance
- improved posture and co-ordination.

Principles of strength and power training

As previously stated, muscular strength can be described as *the amount of force a muscle or muscle group can exert against a resistance*. Power is this force multiplied by velocity. Power activities therefore involve explosive action and may be seen in many athletic activities of short duration such as sprinting, throwing, jumping, lifting, gymnastics, boxing, wrestling, fencing, swimming and cycling.

It has been known for a very long time that strength and power can be significantly improved by training based on an *overload* principle (*see* page 12), and that programmes specifically designed for muscle and muscle group requirements as related to skill will achieve such improvement.

Resistance training is based upon the principles of:
● overload (progressive resistance)
● progression (increase in work)
● specificity (selection of muscles for special overload based on skill and technique).

Muscle loading

Muscles are loaded by performing movements against resistance to maximal muscular contraction. This greatly improves strength and is referred to as working to *repetition maximum* (RM) against a selected resistance.

Maintaining strict exercise technique and working to failure, the following effects may be expected:

● repetitions from 1–6 RM produce strength
● repetitions from 1–6 RM with speed produce power
● repetitions from 7–14 RM produce muscular endurance
● repetitions greater than 15 RM produce stamina.

Working to repetition maximum in this way is known as *overloading* the muscles.

Progressive resistance

As the demands on the body systems are increased, the body moves into a state of *adaptation*. This simply means that more of its resources are challenged to accommodate the increased workload.

An increase in the *quantity* of the overload will cause improved adaptations in the body's levels of endurance and stamina (lighter weights, more repetitions). An increase in the *intensity* (heavier weights and consequently fewer repetitions) will cause improved adaptations in levels of strength and power.

Sometimes it is necessary to devise training programmes that include both approaches. However, since the use of weight resistance is the method of training, the main objective will be to develop power.

Specificity of exercise selection

Those body parts which are most stressed by the exercise programme will benefit most from the training.

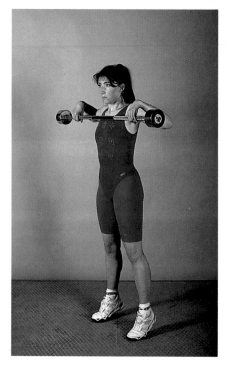

This means that exercises specific to a skill or technique should be included in any workout or training plan. The closer the exercise movement is to the skill of the activity for which the training is designed, the more benefit will be achieved. This will require coaches to have an appropriate sporting knowledge and the ability to analyse movements from both an anatomical and a kinetic perspective.

Reversibility

Any training programme will produce an adaptation of the body systems to the overload placed upon them. However, this adaptation is reversible. To avoid losing the training benefit, the programme should be not only progressive but also continuous, avoiding long periods of rest.

When an athlete first starts to train, it is common for his performance to deteriorate initially; this is because it takes time for the body systems to adapt to the overload which is being applied. Don't lose heart at this stage – keep training and work hard through this difficult period.

Kinetics

In order to understand how to select the appropriate weight training exercises for your particular sport, it is important to have a good knowledge of the actions performed and work done by muscles or groups of muscles. This is the study of *kinetics* and is closely related to the muscular and skeletal anatomy of the body and to the range of movement of levers about the joints.

The skeleton is the framework of the body, both supportive and protective of its vital delicate organs. The skeleton also provides a complex system of levers which conform to the laws of mechanics. The long bones turn about the joints, which act as fulcrums. The muscles contract, acting upon the levers in order to exert force. The greater the resistance to be overcome, the greater the force necessary. This 'force potential' is trainable.

Muscle work

When a muscle contracts it can shorten, lengthen under control, or maintain a fixed position, depending on the load that it is working against.

Concentric contraction

This is when the muscle/muscles actively shorten against a resistance. The muscle attachments move closer together and the joint angle decreases. A good example of this is when performing the two-hand curl with barbell (*see* page 23). The barbell is brought from the front of the thighs to the top of the chest. The flexor muscles of the elbow shorten, developing tension and moving the weight. This is the positive action which constitutes nearly all isotronic weight training exercises.

Eccentric contraction

This is where muscles actively return to their original resting length. As this occurs the muscle develops tension. For example, in the lowering of the bar back to the starting position in the curl, the action of gravity is being controlled. The muscles which contracted concentrically (elbow flexors) are now working eccentrically to control the lowering of the bar.

Static contraction

A muscle or muscle group which is working to maintain a fixed position is said to be working *isometrically* (*iso* = same, *metric* = length). Tension is developed, but there is no resulting movement. Because the tension of the muscle exactly counterbalances the external force, isometric contraction occurs in all sports involving resistance against an external force. Examples include wrestling, judo and gymnastics. Muscles working isometrically also act as stabilisers, 'fixing' a position so that other muscle groups can function concentrically and eccentrically.

Isokinetic contraction

As isometric meant *iso* = same, *metric* = length, so isokinetic means *iso* = same, *kinetic* = motion. When a muscle group contracts it moves a lever through ranges of movement. Some of these ranges are easier to pass through than others. This means that in order to complete the movement, the tension within the muscles is not constant and that consequently any muscle is only working at full force for part of the movement.

In order to fully overload the muscle, exercises and exercise machines have been developed which automatically increase the resistance in the 'easy' parts of the movement. Machines working over cams, levers, hydraulic systems and other mechanical devices automatically change the resistance load on the working muscles and thereby maintain the same degree of muscular tension throughout the full range of movement. This means that resistance is increased at those points where muscle groups are working at their strongest and decreased at those points where the muscles are having to work at positions of mechanical disadvantage. These types of machines were first devised to assist in swimming, where the nature of the resistance provided by the water necessitates movements which maintain speed throughout the action.

Muscle action

Muscles contracting under the various principles described above are also performing *actions*. Here we are concerned with whether the muscle or muscle groups are responsible for the prime movement or for assisting or fixing parts of the body.

Prime movers

These are the muscles which produce the movement. In the curl, the muscles which flex the elbow joint are the prime movers. These are also known as *agonists*.

Antagonists

These are the muscles which would cause the opposite action to the prime movers. When, for example, the flexors of the elbow joint act in the curl, the muscle which lies on the opposite side of the joint would be the antagonist. It will lengthen to permit the elbow to bend under the principle of *reciprocal innervation*. This permits smooth, controlled movement.

Fixators

These muscles will fix a joint or joints so that no movement takes place. They are said to be working *statically* (*see* page 7). A good example of this is seen in bent-forward rowing. Here the muscles of the legs, hips and back are working statically to fix the body in the bent-forward position, whilst the muscles of the shoulder, upper back and arms pull the bar up to the chest and return it to the starting position under control.

Range of movement

Normal healthy muscle activity provides the ability to work from full extension to full flexion of a joint. In doing this the lever is moved through various ranges. This means that there are relatively easy and hard ranges of movement in exercises; many advanced exercises seek to place greater resistance on the harder ranges or, by changing position, make those ranges that are normally easier more difficult to work through. A good example of this is the triceps kickback (bent-forward triceps extension): here,

the greatest possible resistance is placed upon the inner range of the contraction.

Outer range

This is the range at which the muscles are working at their greatest length. At the start of all major isotonic exercises, the muscles pass through this initial range of movement – for example, as the bar is moved from the shoulders in the press and from the front of the thighs in the curl.

Middle range

This is the mid-range of all movements. It is at this stage that the greatest difficulty is often encountered, because although the angle of pull of the muscle is favourable, this is outweighed by the fact that the leverage is at its greatest. Sometimes the weight cannot be moved through this range – this is called the *sticking point*. Additional problems often occur as one group of muscles takes over from another. This means that there is both a mechanical and an anatomical disadvantage to be overcome.

Inner range

This is the range in which the last third of a movement occurs – when the muscle approaches full contraction. It is believed that there is great potential for muscle development at this point, because the muscle must overcome the greatest resistance in this range. That is why advanced exercises such as the triceps kickback, bent-forward curls and hard-lock squats place greatest overload on this inner range.

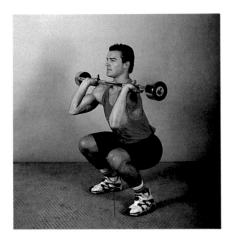

Differences between the physically fit and unfit

In order to understand the reasons why an individual should undergo fitness training, the following comparison between physically fit and unfit persons should be studied.

For easy work that both can sustain in a steady state:

	Fit	Unfit
● Oxygen consumption	Lower	Higher
● Pulse rate during work	Lower	Higher
● Stroke volume during work	Larger	Smaller
● Blood pressure during work	Lower	Higher
● Blood lactate	Lower	Higher
● Return of blood pressure to normal after work	Faster	Slower
● Return of pulse rate to resting value after work	Faster	Slower

For exhausting work that neither can sustain in a steady state:

	Fit	Unfit
● Maximum oxygen consumption	Higher	Lower
● Maximum pulse rate during work	Usually Lower	Usually Higher
● Stroke volume	Larger	Smaller
● Duration of work before exhaustion	Longer	Shorter
● Return of blood pressure to normal after work	Faster	Slower
● Return of pulse rate to resting value after work	Faster	Slower

Summary of main benefits of fitness

There are many benefits of physical fitness. They include:

- improved muscle tone
- increased agility
- improved mechanical efficiency
- improved capacity for relaxation
- increased ability for concentration during training and competition
- improved metabolic, physiological and possibly psychological efficiency. Blood pressure is decreased and heart and breathing rates lowered
- sport performance can increase because a greater degree of fatigue can be endured and recovery is quicker
- general feeling of well-being.

Attainment of fitness involves a change of physiological state with improved efficiency. The process takes time and cannot be achieved in a few training sessions. In practice, a good deal of time is given over to cardio-vascular and other fitness work in the early part of the training period.

Physical fitness terminology

- **Aerobic training** is used for the improvement of general endurance. The training effort varies from moderate to high intensity. With aerobic training the athlete has sufficient oxygen for his output. The greater the cardio-vascular reserve of the athlete, the higher is his aerobic capacity.

- **Anaerobic training** is characterised by efforts of maximal or submaximal intensity whereby sufficient oxygen is not available for the athlete's neuromuscular output. The anaerobic performance lasts for a few seconds (or less, as in speed or strength performances). The aerobic effort depends on the athlete's capacity to tolerate the 'oxygen debt' (s.q.) involved. This type of training is necessary for the development of muscular energy.

- **Steady state** is the term used when the athlete's oxygen intake and consumption are kept at a steady level with waste product being oxydised as they occur.

- **Oxygen debt.** In performances involving bursts of great strength or speed, the oxygen intake is insufficient to meet the demands of the body. The athlete is said to incur an *oxygen debt*. In some cases less than 25% of the inhaled oxygen passes into the blood and the working muscles. Excess fatigue products, principally lactic acid, are produced and spill over into the blood by 'buffering reactions'. In the recovery phase after the intense activity these fatigue products are oxydised, or in more common terms the oxygen debt is repaid. It is possible to reach such a high level of lactic acid such that the muscle can no longer contract, thereby limiting performance. Thus it follows that athletes need to develop a high oxygen debt tolerance.

Warm-up

Vital capacity of the lungs is the largest quantity of air a person can forcibly expel from his lungs after the deepest inhalation possible. It is sometimes known as Forced Vital Capacity (FVC). Vital capacity is thought to be closely related to body weight and body surface area. In addition there is evidence to suggest that there is a relationship between physical work and vital capacity. The ratio FEV 1 sec./FVC (Forced Expiratory Volume at 1 second divided by Forced Vital Capacity) is a useful measure of lung efficiency.

Before exercising with weights, the athlete should perform some gentle exercises to prepare for the more vigorous activity to come. These exercises will be free standing, and as well as preparing the cardio-vascular and circulo-respiratory systems for activity by light aerobic work, should pay careful attention to full-range flexibility work for all the major joints on which the principal muscle groups will act in the weight training movements.

The warm-up therefore fulfils the following functions.

- It takes the athlete gradually from the demands of daily activity to the increased pressures on body systems that sport and training require.
- For those involved in sport, it creates an opportunity to rehearse – both physically and mentally – the techniques of the activity.
- It increases the body temperature.
- It increases the supply of oxygen in the tissues.
- It improves the removal of waste products of exercise.
- It improves reaction time.
- It helps to reduce the chances of injury.

Always warm up and taper down.

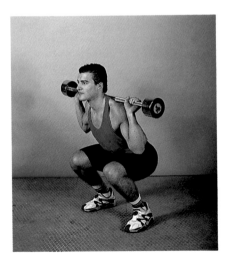

Breathing

With few exceptions it is advisable to breathe *in* whilst *lifting* the weight and *out* whilst *lowering* it. For beginners, this advice is especially important as it gives a rhythm to the movement and prevents a tendency to hold the breath for several repetitions.

By breathing in as we perform movements on a repetition basis we make a solid base for the muscles to work from. Once you understand the anatomy of the exercises you will be able to work out the breathing for yourself. However, this book gives clear recommendations for beginners and for less experienced athletes.

There are some exceptions to the above rule; these are described in the exercise rubric. Such variations apply when the trunk is flexed, as in the abdominal exercises when the action of sitting up forces the air out. Also, in rib expanding exercises where the spine is extended and the ribs are elevated – such as the pullover and flying exercises – the breathing action is *in* as the weights are *lowered*, thereby taking advantage of the stretching action of the movement.

These recommendations apply to movements where the resistance is such that 8–10 or more repetitions can be performed. In maximum attempts, or where records are being performed, the lifters will take a deep breath and hold it whilst performing the lift. They then breathe out at the conclusion of the movement. Generally, such attempts create great strain and are undertaken only within the area of Olympic or powerlifting competition and in some forms of very heavy advanced weight training.

Overload

The concept of overload is generally seen as referring to an increase in weight handled. To achieve this progressively, heavier weights are used for each exercise.

Overload can, however, be applied in various ways as follows:

● **muscle overload** – progressive resistance, increase in weight handled

● **systematic overload** – overload in other body systems, such as cardio-vascular, circulo-respiratory. Such overload is brought about by: increased repetition; increased sets of repetitions; decrease in time taken for exercise between sets and exercise; increase in time taken extending bouts of exercise; increase in frequency of exercising.

Let us see how this may work.

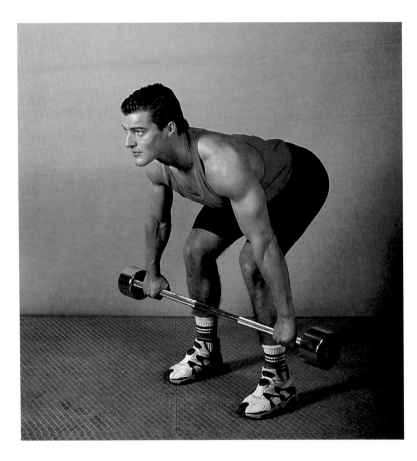

Example

The subject is a beginner in poor physical condition, possibly middle-aged and having done little exercise for some years. The type of training loads followed by the fit, athletic young person will be entirely inappropriate to such an individual. However, in order to provide the necessary fitness programme to cater for systematic rehabilitation, we must follow a training regime that will employ the overload principle. Programmes may therefore be arranged on the following basis.

Schedule A

Objectives
- Learn the exercise skills (major large muscle group movement).
- Develop fitness – increase muscle rate.
- Duration – 4–6 weeks.
- Frequency – three times per week (Mon, Wed, Fri).

Exercise	Weight	Sets	Reps 2 weeks	Reps 2–4 weeks	Reps 4–6 weeks
High pull up	Token	1	10	12	14
Press from chest	Token	1	10	12	14
Two-hand curl	Token	1	10	12	14
Upright rowing	Token	1	10	12	14
Bench press	Token	1	10	12	14
Back half squat (progressing to full squat)	Token	1	10	12	14
Straight-arm pullovers (progressive)	Token	1	10	12	14
Dumb-bell side bends	Token	1	10	12	14
Gentle abdominal (progressive)	Token	1	10	12	14

At the end of six weeks the lifter should be performing 14 reps for each exercise so that the last three or four reps are hard work but are performed (as with all other reps) under the principle of 'strict exercise technique'. This method of building up the repetitions is an overload on the cardio-vascular and circulo-respiratory system.

Having achieved these repetition maximums, the weight can now be increased. Based upon observations of the performance of the lifter and his size and progress, the coach will make the appropriate selection of weight increase. This is *progressive resistance* (*see* page 5). The repetitions are then built up in precisely the same way until the desired maximum is again reached and then the weight can be increased again. This type of training can continue indefinitely since this method of overload – through repetition increase – focuses the work on those systems concerned with heart and lung improvement in addition to muscular strength training.

Whilst great muscular strength is not the objective in itself, improvements will be made since the increase in weight being loaded for each exercise at the beginning of each period of six weeks will provide muscular overload.

Schedule B

As the lifter improves, he will feel the need to do more work and so a second set of each exercise will be appropriate. The lifter is now working for two sets of the required build-up of repetitions with increased weight. *The overload demands are increasing.* It may be argued that such a schedule will become boring, but since these exercises cater for the major muscle groups of the body, change is not necessary as such. A variation of schedule is wise, however. The exercises are still very similar, but the trainer will sense a change in emphasis.

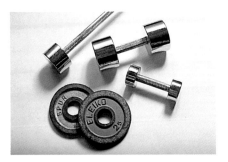

Exercise	Weight	Sets	Reps 2 weeks	Reps 2–4 weeks	Reps 4–6 weeks
Power clean	According to progress	2	10	12	14
Press behind neck or dumb-bell press	"	2	10	12	14
Dumb-bell curls	"	2	10	12	14
Bent-over rowing	"	2	10	12	14
Dumb-bell flying (Pec Deck machine)	"	2	10	12	14
Front squat	"	2	10	12	14
Bent arm pullover	"	2	10	12	14
Twisting single arm rowing (each side)	"	2	10	12	14
Abdominals	"	2	10	12	14

Since we now have two schedules of exercise (very similar in effect for the muscle group being exercised but giving a variation in exercise technique), the lifter can further increase the training load by increasing the frequency of the number of training sessions per week – for instance to four times per week as follows:

Mon	Tues	Wed	Thurs	Fri	Sat	Sun
Schedule A	Schedule B	Rest	Schedule A	Schedule B	Light aerobic exercise	Rest

(Schedule A is increased to two sets for each exercise.)

The fact that schedules follow each other over a two-day work plan challenges the body systems to accept the stimulation of repeated overload. This is a very effective method of achieving fitness, especially in an aerobic capacity. Many people believe that the overload method works only on the muscular system, with little advantage to be gained for the cardio-vascular/circulo-respiratory system. This is not so as long as rests between sets do not exceed 90 seconds. Indeed, such rest periods of 60–90 sec. should apply to all types of progressive resistance training.

Power development

For our purpose it is correct to conceive power as a combination of strength and speed (Force × Velocity). Strength can be seen as a raw quality in which a maximum force is applied for a very short period of time. Activities such as bending iron bars, tearing telephone directories in half and dinamometric activities where the muscular contraction is isometric are examples of this.

When a resistance is selected that will permit high levels of strength to be demonstrated isotonically, at maximum speed as permitted by the resistance, the trainer will be developing *power*. Highly dynamic performances that last for comparatively short periods of time therefore demonstrate power production. Whilst activities such as sprinting, throwing, jumping and Olympic lifting may look totally different in performance, the essential qualities of strength and speed (power) are the same and therefore, excluding the technique-specific elements of the activity, many of the training requirements will be the same.

In Olympic weightlifting, the snatch and clean and jerk, where weights up to three times the athlete's bodyweight are lifted, enormous amounts of power must be generated. The lifter must therefore be very strong and very fast-moving. Experience has shown that this high level of power will only be developed when handling weights of 70% and above, with the more experienced lifting 80% and above. This means that if a lifter can snatch 150 kg at 81 kg bodyweight (the old 'light heavy' class), he will only make significant training developments if the greater part of his training is completed with weights in the range of 120 kg and above for this lift. Training loadings will therefore be based upon heavy weights and of course consequently lower repetitions. Weightlifters will therefore rarely do more than five repetitions in a set, and more usually perform threes, twos and singles. Weights lighter than 70% are regarded as having value for warm-up, skills rehearsal and fitness training only.

However, it is correct to point out that in many sports, whilst the requirement is based upon power and because the activity goes on for long periods of time, *endurance* is also of prime importance. Training for these power endurance sports (for example, rowing, canoeing, tennis and cycling) can be greatly enhanced by including programmes of power training throughout the season. Initially the exercises are of a massive major muscle group design and repetitions are high (between 10 and 15) with a resistance that will permit the final three or four reps to be performed with great determination but employing the principles of strict exercise technique. As the trainer becomes accustomed to the performance and loading of the major muscle group exercises, then specific exercises can be introduced into the schedules. These exercises are based upon the critical power expression points of the activity and require that the coach has basic understanding of the sport technique and the anatomy and kinetics of the performance.

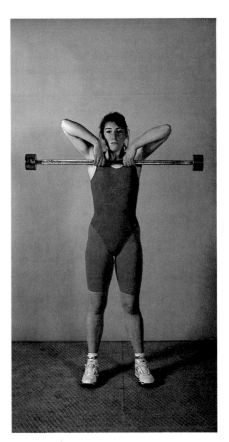

Warming up

Before any weight training it is essential that you follow a short warm-up period of free standing exercises. These should include full range mobility work for all the major joint complexes of the body.

Exercise
Get set or starting position.

Body part developed
This is the basic lifting position for all lifts. The emphasis is on legs and hips and a strong, flat back.

Performance/action
Feet hip-width apart. The weight of the body is over all of the foot. Bending the legs and hips, grasp the bar. Keep the back flat and strong and the arms straight. Drive strongly with the legs and stand erect.

Breathing
Breathe in as you lift the bar and out as you return to the starting position.

Recommendations
This is the basic lifting technique. It is a life skill. Use the strong muscles of the legs and hips to overcome the resistance. This skill must be learnt first to eliminate the possibility of injuries to the back that can so easily result from incorrect lifting procedures.

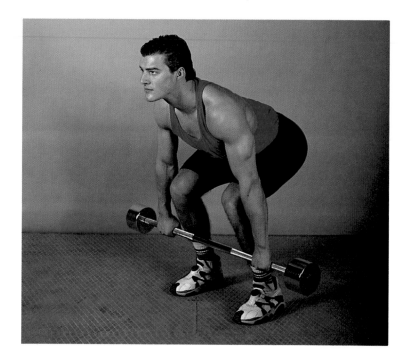

Exercise
High pull-up.

Body part developed
With light weights this is an ideal warm-up exercise. With heavier resistance it is a great power builder.

Performance/action
From the starting position, drive with the legs. Lift the bar high, keeping the chest up. Note that the elbows are above the bar and the lifter rises high up on the toes.

Breathing
Breathe in as you lift the bar and out as you lower back to the starting position.

Recommendations
Make the exercise rhythmic. Keep the chest up and do not dip down to the bar.

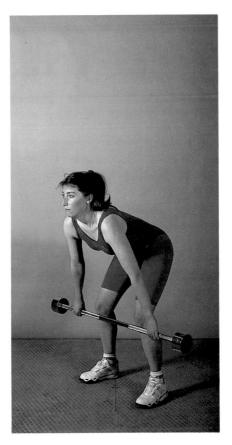

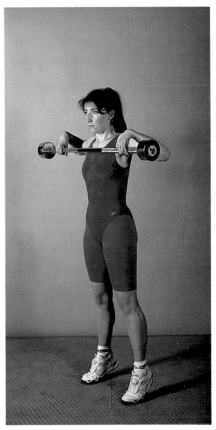

Exercise
Power clean with bar-bell.

Body part developed
This is one of the most important all-round power builders affecting all the major muscle groups.

Performance/action
From the starting position, drive strongly with the legs and vigorously extend the back. Bring the arms into action as the bar-bell passes the mid-thighs. Catch the bar up on the shoulders and keep the elbows high. Dip the legs slightly as you receive the bar.

Breathing
Breathe in as you lift and out as you lower back to the starting position. When this exercise is performed for repetitions, it can have a very positive effect on the cardio-vascular system.

Recommendations
After you have received the bar on the chest, lower it first to the thighs then, keeping the back flat, return to the starting position and bend the legs.

Variations
This exercise can be performed with dumb-bells.

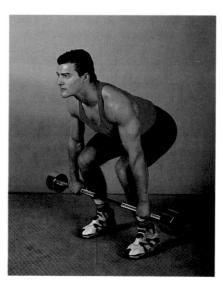

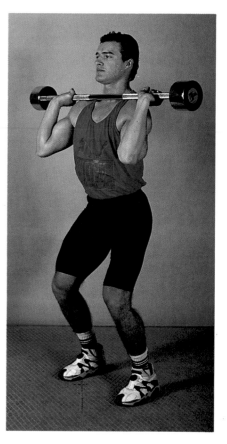

Exercise
Upright rowing.

Body part developed
The muscles of the shoulders and upper back as well as the muscles which flex the elbow joint.

Performance/action
From the starting position, pull the bar up to the chin, keeping the elbows higher than the bar.

Breathing
Breathe in as the bar is lifted and out as you return it to the starting position.

Recommendations
The bar should be gripped centrally with the hands about 6 inches apart, knuckles to the front. Lower the bar under control.

Variations
With heavier weights the more advanced trainer may use the legs slightly to get the bar moving through the outer range.

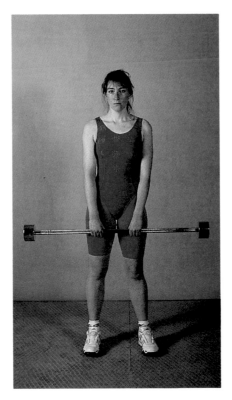
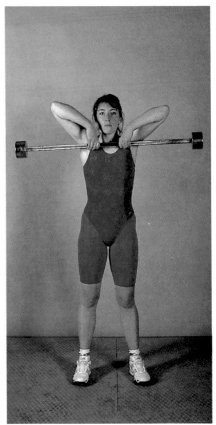

Exercise
Press behind neck.

Body part developed
The muscles of the shoulders and the back of the upper arm.

Performance/action
From the position with the bar resting on the rear shoulders, head set slightly forward, press the bar straight to arms' length over the head.

Breathing
Breathe in as the bar is pressed upwards and out as it is lowered back to the shoulders, under control.

Recommendations
The bar should be power cleaned to the front of the shoulders. Then, with a little dip, it should be taken over the head on to the shoulders behind the head. The grip can then be widened slightly for comfort.

Variations
This exercise can be performed from the front of the chest.

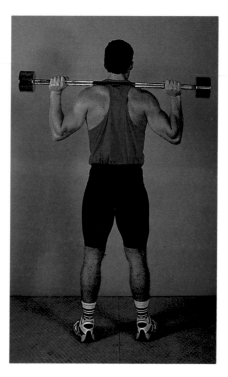

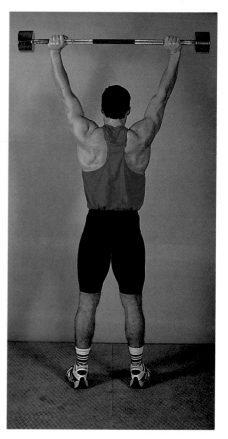

Exercise
Two-hands curl with bar-bell.

Body part developed
The muscles on the front of the upper arm which flex the elbow joint.

Performance/action
Making sure that the bar-bell is kept close to the body throughout the movement, curl the bar to the top of the chest.

Breathing
Breathe in as the bar is raised and out as it is returned to the starting position under control.

Recommendations
When performing the exercise the elbows must remain behind the bar and be free from the sides of the body. This will mean that the greater resistance will be on the muscles on the inner range of the action.

Variations
There are many variations of this exercise with bar-bells, dumb-bells and machines. By varying the width of grip or changing the position of the body, the effect of the resistance can be changed.

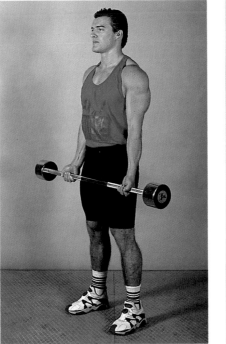
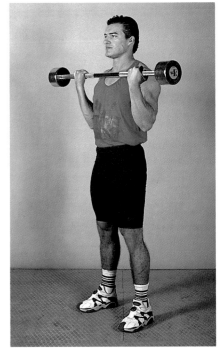

Exercise
Bent forward rowing.

Body part developed
The upper back muscles and the flexors of the elbow.

Performance/action
From the starting position, the bar-bell is pulled strongly up to the chest by bending the arms and raising the elbows sideways. This is an excellent exercise for improving posture.

Breathing
Breathe in as the bar is pulled up to the chest and out as it is lowered back to the starting position.

Recommendations
Note that the body remains still throughout the movement. The legs are slightly bent at the knees. This relieves pressure on the muscles at the rear of the legs (hamstrings) in this bent forward position.

Variations
By pulling the bar to various parts of the trunk, the effect can be varied. For instance, if the bar is pulled to the abdomen, the lower part of the back is principally exercised.

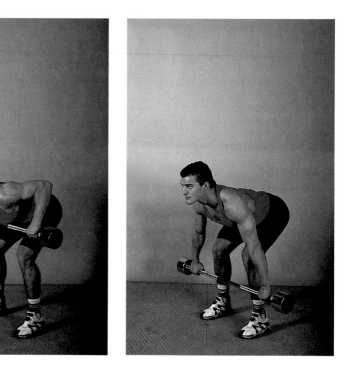

Exercise
Back squat (deep knee bend).

Body part developed
Develops power in the legs, hips, back and chest. Improves the condition of the lungs and heart.

Performance/action
From the starting position with the bar resting on the shoulder behind the head, lower the body by bending at the knees and hips. Keep the feet flat on the floor. Beginners may use a slight elevation under the heels, but as ankle mobility improves this should soon be discontinued. Keep the knees pointing out throughout the movement. From the low position, thighs parallel, keep the head up, at the same time strongly driving with the legs to rise.

Breathing
For repetition squats fill the lungs with air, bend the legs, breathe out just as you hit the low position, and breathe in as you rise. As very heavy weights can be used in this exercise, single maximum attempts will require the lifter to take a breath, lower and rise breathing out at the conclusion of the movement.

Recommendations
The back squat is one of the most important power development exercises, and fairly rapid progress can be made. Due to the large groups of major muscles being used, great demands are made on the circulatory and respiratory systems. This exercise greatly encourages increase in muscular body weight.

Variations
There are many leg exercises which are all variations of the squat. These range from step-ups with weights, to lunges, and squat or vertical jumps.

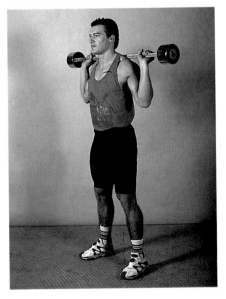
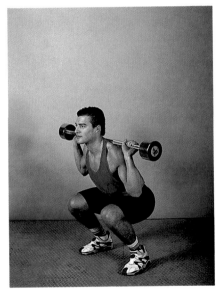

Exercise
Front squat.

Body part developed
Because of the upright position of the trunk with the bar held on the chest, the resistance is thrown more directly on to the muscles on the front of the thighs and the hip muscles.

Performance/action
Place the feet hip-width apart with the bar on the top of the chest. Lower the body to the squat position. Drive upwards vigorously. Keep the elbows high throughout the action.

Breathing
Take a breath. Breathe out as you lower and in as you rise to the standing position. Repeat this action with the rhythm of the movement.

Recommendations
Keep the knees out as you squat and rise.

Variations
All leg exercises are variations of squat movements.

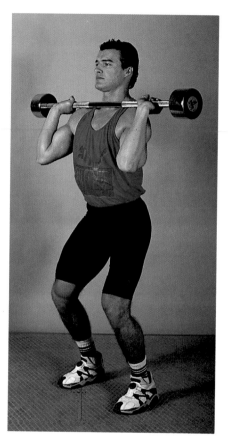
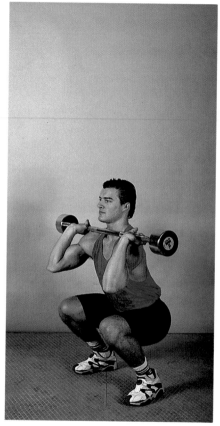

Exercise
French press – standing triceps press with dumb-bell.

Body part developed
The muscles at the rear of the upper arm.

Performance/action
Stand with the body well braced, feet hip-width apart. Lower the dumb-bell to behind the head. From this position, vigorously extend the elbow until the dumb-bell is above the shoulder.

Breathing
Breathe in on the effort of raising the dumb-bell, and out as it is lowered.

Recommendations
Exercise each arm for sets alternately. Use the opposite hand to hold the upper arm to stabilise the base for the movement.

Variations
All triceps exercises have a similar effect.

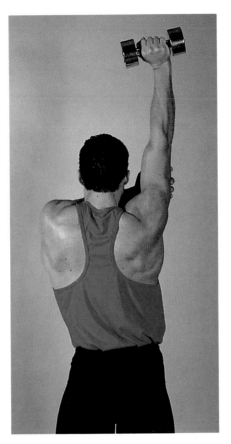
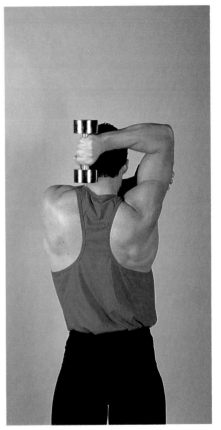

Exercise
Bent forward triceps press with dumb-bells (triceps kickbacks).

Body part developed
This exercise has a very strong effect on the development of the muscles on the back of the upper arms.

Performance/action
With the feet astride and the knees slightly bent, incline the trunk forwards. Keep the elbows pointing upwards with the inside of the upper arms held firmly against the sides of the trunk and the dumb-bell hanging below the shoulders. Extend the elbows. Keep the body, shoulders and upper arms still during this movement.

Breathing
Breathe in as the elbows are extended.

Recommendations
This is a long lever exercise where the greatest resistance is thrown on the inner range of the muscles' contraction. It is an advanced exercise. At each extension hold the position for a fraction of a second. This greatly enhances the exercise effect.

Variations
All triceps exercises – though most are not as advanced as this.

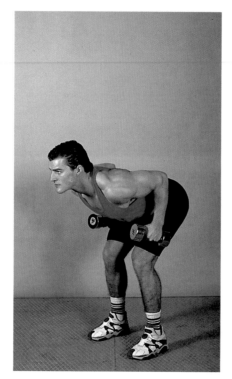

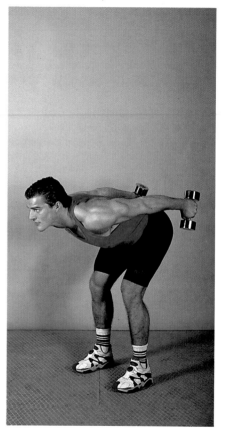

Exercise
Dumb-bell screw curl.

Body part developed
This exercise is specially designed to develop the biceps, which is responsible for *supination* of the hand (i.e. the twisting motion at the elbow which turns the hand upwards). The biceps is greatly assisted by the brachialis in elbow flexion.

Performance/action
Stand erect, feet hip-width apart. The dumb-bell should be held at the sides pointing fore and aft. Bend the arms strongly; as the bells pass through the mid-position they should be turned so that they lie across the body at the conclusion of the movement. Reverse the movement to return the bells to the starting position. Do not allow the elbows to come too far forwards so that the resistance is kept on the muscles.

Breathing
Breathe in as the dumb-bells are curled and out as they are returned to the starting position.

Recommendations
Keep the elbows back to maintain maximum resistance on the inner range of the contraction.

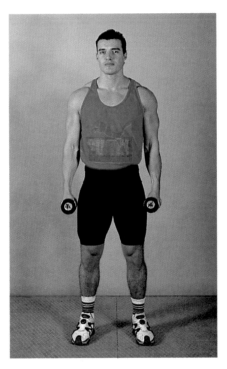
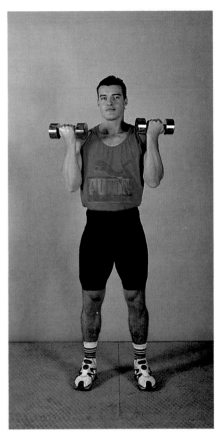

Exercise
Bent forward lateral raise.

Body part developed
To develop the abductors of the shoulder blades and the muscles which cap the posterior of the shoulder joint.

Performance/action
Feet hip-width apart, knees unlocked, trunk inclined forwards, back flat. The dumb-bells are held at arms' length beneath the shoulders. Maintaining the starting position, raise the dumb-bells sideways to a point slightly above the shoulder joints.

Breathing
Breathe in as the dumb-bells are raised and out as they are lowered under control back to the starting position.

Variations
This exercise can be performed with pulley machines.

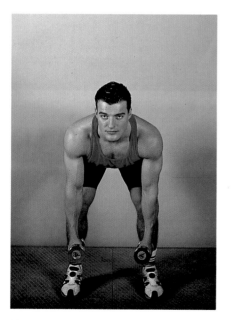 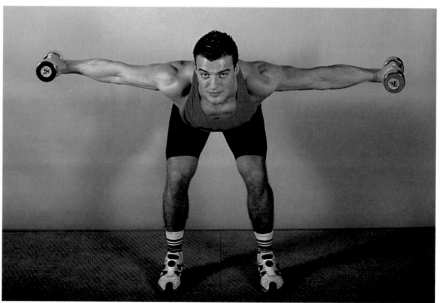

Exercise
Lateral raise standing with dumb-bells.

Body part developed
To develop the muscles of the shoulders and upper back, especially the middle portion of the deltoid muscle which caps the shoulder.

Performance/action
Stand with the feet hip-width apart, body upright and dumb-bells held at your sides. Raise the dumb-bells sideways. Raise the chest at the same time. Lower back to the starting position – repeat.

Breathing
Breathe in as the bells are raised and out as they are lowered under control to the starting position.

Variations
This exercise can be performed with pulley machines.

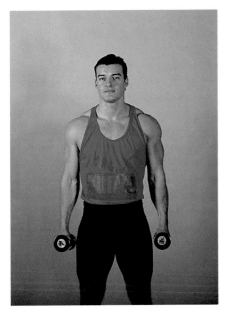
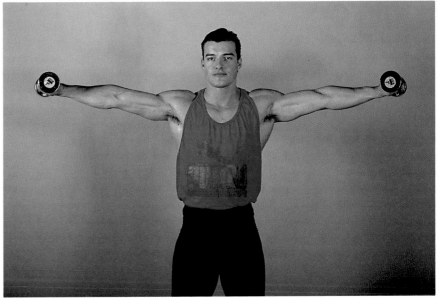

Exercise
Dumb-bell press.

Body part developed
Muscles of the shoulders, backs of the upper arms and upper back muscles.

Performance/action
Feet hip-width apart, body erect and firmly braced. With a dumb-bell in each hand bring them to the shoulders. From this position press the bells evenly to arms' length over the head.

Breathing
Breathe in as you press the bells to arms' length and out as you lower them back to the starting position under control.

Recommendations
Lift the chest as you press the dumb-bells. Dumb-bell work has a very positive strengthening effect; this is especially true of overhead exercises, as the bells are much more difficult to control than a bar-bell.

Variations
All pressing actions with free weights and machines will have similar effect. Can also be performed seated.

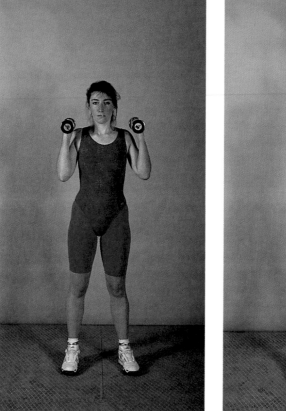
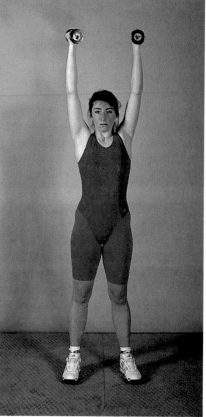

Exercise
Dumb-bell side bend.

Body part developed
Muscles on the side of the trunk.

Performance/action
Stand with the feet well apart with the dumb-bell in one hand. Lean over to the side of the dumb-bell. Place the opposite hand behind the head. Maintain a lateral plane of movement by pushing the hips forwards slightly. Now bend the body strongly against the resistance. Keep the arm straight. Don't try to lift the dumb-bell. Keep the feet flat on the floor.

Breathing
Breath in as you raise the weight and out as you return to the starting position.

Recommendations
Make sure that you exercise over the fullest range of movement. The exercise is for the trunk muscles on the opposite side to the dumb-bell. When you have completed the required number of repetitions for one side, change hands and repeat on the opposite side.

Variations
Can be performed with pulley machines.

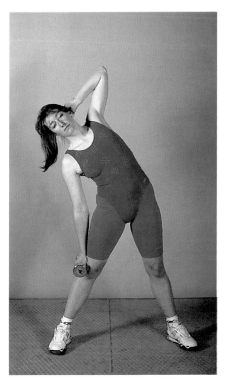

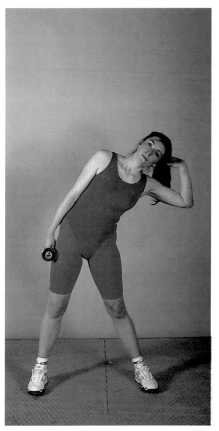

33

Exercise
Forward raise standing with dumb-bells.

Body part developed
To develop the muscles on the front of the shoulders.

Performance/action
Feet hip-width apart with the body upright. The dumb-bells rest across the front of the thighs. Keeping the arms straight, raise the dumb-bells forwards to a point slightly above the level of the shoulders. Keep the chest high throughout the movement.

Breathing
Breathe in on the effort of raising the dumb-bells and out as they are lowered under control back to the starting position.

Variations
Similar exercises can be performed with pulley machines.

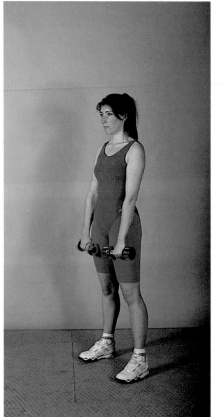
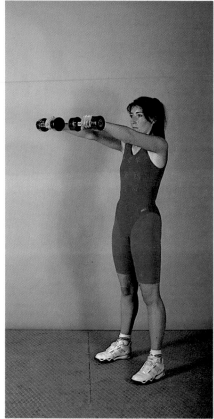

Exercise
Press on bench.

Body part developed
To develop the muscles on the front of the chest and shoulders, the side of the trunk and the muscles on the back of the upper arms.

Performance/action
For the beginner the starting position is with the bar resting on the chest. This ensures that the exercise is safe. Lie on the bench, knees bent and feet flat on the floor for stability. The bar is passed to you by two assistants who help lower it until it rests on the chest. When you feel confident and comfortable say 'my bar' and the assistants will release it. They must however stand ready at all times to give assistance if needed. From this position the bar is pressed to arms' length above the chest. Lower the bar back to the starting position, with assistance if necessary, and repeat.

Breathing
Breathe in as the bar is pressed up, and out as it is returned to the chest under control.

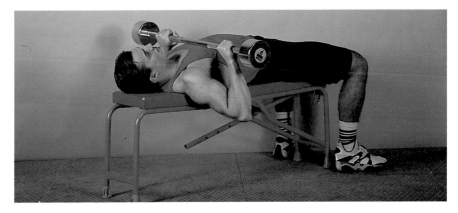

Recommendations
This is a major exercise and is a competition lift in the sport of powerlifting. Under those conditions the bar is taken from stands and part of the lift is to lower it to the chest before pressing it. The breathing is then different, as a full breath of air is taken in before the bar is lifted from the stands. This is held until the conclusion of the lift when the bar is at arms' length. Never train alone on this lift.

Variations
There are many variations on this

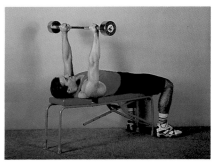

exercise. The bench can be inclined or declined and different grip widths can be used. Dumb-bells and machines.

Exercise
Single arm rowing with trunk rotation. (Can also be performed without trunk rotation.)

Body part developed
To develop the muscles which rotate the trunk, shoulders and upper back, and the muscles which flex the elbow.

Performance/action
Take a comfortable feet-astride position with one hand resting on a low bench and the dumb-bell in the other hand at arms' length. The dumb-bell is pulled vigorously upwards to the shoulder whilst rotating the trunk.

Breathing
Breathe in as the dumb-bell is raised and out as it and the trunk are returned to the starting position.

Recommendations
This is a very important exercise for trunk rotation. Remember that this rotating action can only be performed against gravity if it is to have the desired effect.

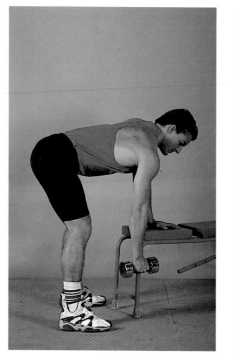
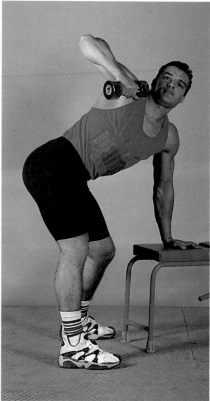

Exercise
Straight-arm pullover.

Body part developed
To enlarge the thorax and develop the muscles surrounding the shoulder girdle, front of the chest and the large muscles of the lower back.

Performance/action
Lie on the bench with the feet firmly on the ground and the bar at arms' length above the shoulders. Keeping the arms straight, lower the bar until the arms are horizontal to the floor. Then pull the bar back to the position above the chest.

Breathing
As this exercise expands the rib-cage the action is enhanced by breathing in as the bar is lowered. Breathe out at it is pulled back to the starting position above the shoulders.

Recommendations
As this is a long lever movement, care must be taken. Lower the barbell slowly and over a steadily increasing range of movement to gauge the stretch available from repetition to repetition.

Variations
Can be performed with dumb-bells and on specialised machines.

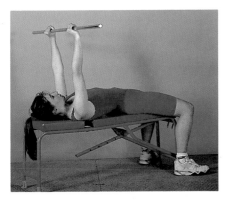

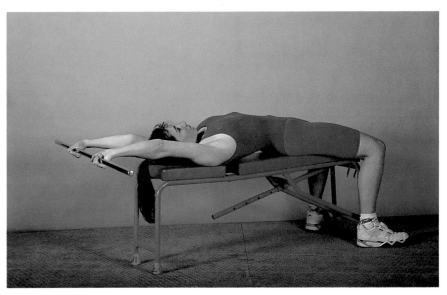

Exercise
Lateral raise lying.

Body part developed
To develop the muscles of the chest and front of the shoulders.

Performance/action
Lying flat on the bench, knees bent and feet flat on the floor for stability. The dumb-bells are held at arms' length vertically above the shoulders. Keeping the arms straight, the dumb-bells are lowered sideways until they are level with the shoulder joints horizontal to the floor.

Breathing
As this exercise helps to expand the rib-cage, breathe in as the bells are lowered and out as they are returned to the starting position.

Recommendations
Train with two supporters using very light dumb-bells to start with. As this is a long lever movement, gradually increase the range of movement with each repetition.

Variations
All rib expansion exercises. The 'Pec Deck'.

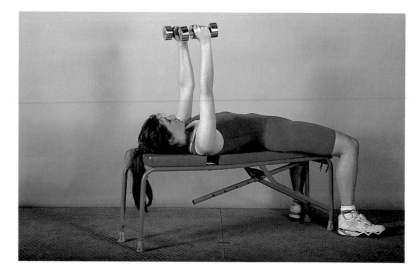

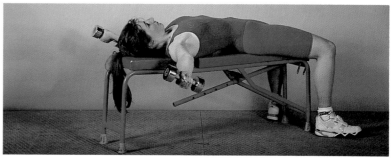

Exercise
Chest press ('Pec Deck').

Body part developed
This exercise develops the muscles of the chest and the front of the shoulders and expands the rib cage.

Performance/action
Keeping the elbows at 90° with the forearms on the pads, bring the forearms together in front of the chest. Sit with the head and back against the back pads.

Breathing
Take a breath then breathe out as the arms are brought together. Breathe in as the arms move apart. Since this is a rib-cage expanding exercise, the action is assisted by these reversed breathing instructions.

Recommendations
Some machines have hand grips. Grasp these firmly. There are also pullover machines which have a similar effect and similar machines in a horizontal position.

Variations
All free weight pullover exercises and lateral raise lying (flying exercise).

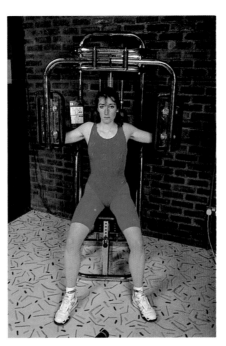
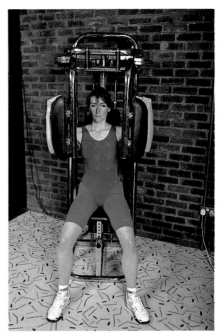

Exercise
Seated 'Lat' pulldowns.

Body part developed
To develop the upper back muscles (*Latissimus dorsi*), and to some extent the muscles on the front of the upper arm.

Performance/action
Sit down with the knees under the pads. Take a fairly wide hand space. Pull the bar down to touch the back of the neck gently. Let the bar return to the starting position under control.

Breathing
Breathe in as the bar is pulled down and out as it is returned to the starting position.

Recommendations
The bar can also be pulled to the front of the chest for a slight variation on the exercise.

Variations
'Chinning' on a bar.

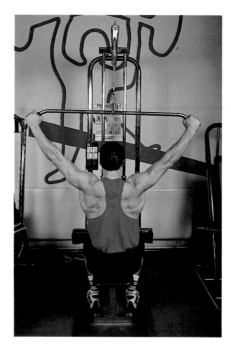
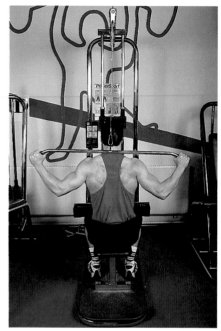

Exercise
Knee extensions.

Body part developed
To develop the muscles on the front of the upper leg (the quadriceps).

Performance/action
Sit on the apparatus with the feet under the pads on the insteps. Hold the handles firmly, body against the back-rest. The legs are fully extended at the knee. Hold the position for a fraction of a second then under control bend the legs and return to the starting position.

Breathing
Breathe in as the legs are extended and out as they return to the starting position.

Recommendations
The seat and backrest positions are usually adjustable – make sure that your position is comfortable and that the leg length lever is correctly adjusted.

Variations
Can be performed with an iron boot.

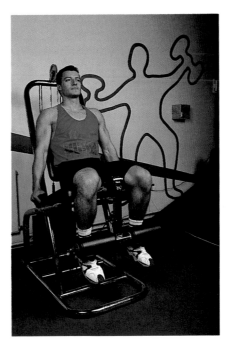
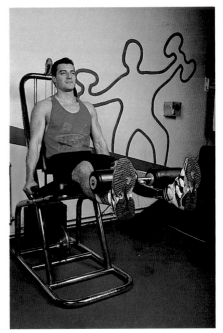

Exercise
Leg curls.

Body part developed
To develop the muscles on the back of the upper leg (hamstrings).

Performance/action
Lie face downwards on the bench. Place the heels under the roller pads. Make sure that all the body is in touch with the bench and grasp the handles firmly. Pull the heels up as far as possible and then, under control, return to the starting position.

Breathing
Breathe in as the curling action of raising the weight is performed and out as the knees straighten.

Recommendations
Adjust the leg lever so that the knees are over the edge of the bench.

Variations
This exercise can be performed with free weight apparatus; this is called an 'iron boot'.

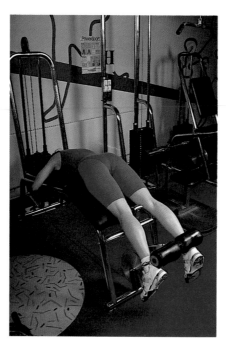
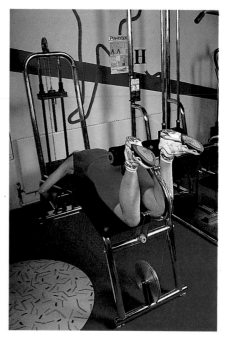

Exercise
Horizontal leg press.

Body part developed
To develop the large muscles on the front of the upper leg and the muscles of the hips.

Performance/action
Sit with your back against the back pad and grip the handles firmly. Place all of the flat of the feet against the pushing foot plate. Extend the legs until the knees are locked. By bending the legs, return the weight to the starting position.

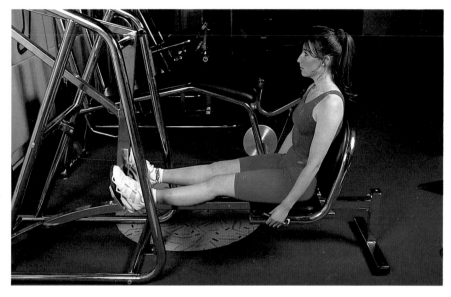

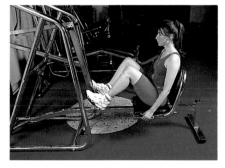

Breathing
Breathe in as the legs are extended and out as they return to the starting position under control.

Recommendations
Before performing the exercise adjust the seat distance from the pushing foot plate so that when in the starting position the angle at the back of the knees is 90°.

Variations
The exercise can be performed on the vertical leg press machine.

Exercise
Graduated abdominal exercise.

Body part developed
Muscles on the front of the abdomen and those which flex the hip joint.

Performance/action
With a partner holding your feet (or using any other method of fixing the feet), lie on the back with the knees bent and the hands resting on the front of the thighs. Slide the hands up to the knees at the same time flexing the trunk. Lower under control, allowing the hands to slide back down the thighs.

Breathing
Breathe in then out as you flex and in as you return to the starting position. Repeat the movement, breathing out as you sit up.

Recommendations
Progress slowly with all abdominal exercises.

Variations
Many variations, all increasing in severity.

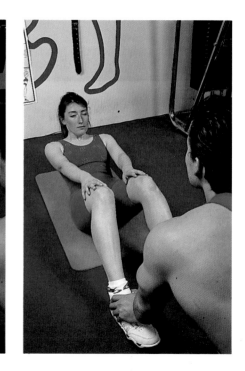

Weightlifting safety

Safety for teachers and coaches

Every coach and teacher wants to prevent accidents. To protect your athletes/pupils and yourself:

General physical education

● Have all equipment inspected regularly. Report in writing all deficiencies in apparatus, mats, floor surfaces, rigs, equipment, etc., to your superior. Don't use until put right. *Get the best equipment and keep it in good condition.*
● Make sure you have taught all the necessary *skills*, including safety procedures, before requiring anyone to exercise them in game, class or competition situations.
● Get medical approval before putting an injured person back into game, class or competition activity.
● Beginners need special teaching and supervision. A champion trying out an entirely new skill is a beginner at that skill. *Supervision means being there when needed.*
● Fatigue often precedes accidents. For the work to be attempted the person must be fit.

Weight training and lifting

In addition to the above, keep the apparatus locked up unless at least three people want to use it.

● Ensure that your layout for the different exercises in the weight training area is carefully planned. Barbells should not be too close to each other. Use mats under the weights. Transport of equipment requires great care. *Do not permit horseplay.*
● Check the barbells, stands, benches, dumb-bells, etc., carefully before use. Make sure all collars are tight and barbells evenly loaded. Check the apparatus each time it comes out and after every set: *it is your responsibility.*

● Only train in an area where the floor is even, firm and non-slip. Do not permit individuals to train in bare feet. *Balance in progressive resistance training is very important.*
● Check and service your equipment regularly: *it's good insurance.*
● Know *why* and *when* to teach specific exercises, as well as *how*. Good intentions are no excuse for ignorance. *Attend an official coaching course.*
● Make sure that stand-ins (two) are used for all exercises, one each side of the barbell ready to assist. Teach all pupils how to stand-in and catch. *Ensure that the stand-in knows when and how to help.*
● Ensure that lifters do not attempt limit poundages too soon. *Too great a weight = bad body position = accident.*
● Teach exercises carefully. Ensure strict exercise principles are employed at all times. *Every pupil must advance at his own level.*
● Use only token resistance during the exercise learning phase. When

muscle groups are weak, they lack control. Lack of muscular control can lead to injury. *Proceed with caution and always with careful supervision.*

● Correct breathing on all lifts must be taught. *Apply correct training principles.*

● Encourage the use of warm clothing in which to train and fast training procedure to avoid local chilling of muscles. *Employ correct training principles.*

● Before driving your lifters on to advanced training schedules or to competitions at too early a stage in their career, analyse your motives. Unless the well-being and safety of the performers come above personal vanity and ambition, it could be a dangerous programme. *Integrity is the keyword to remember when supervising lifters.*

● Display a notice in the gymnasium and ensure that everyone is familiar with the recommendations. Have your rules and enforce them. *Stay in charge.*

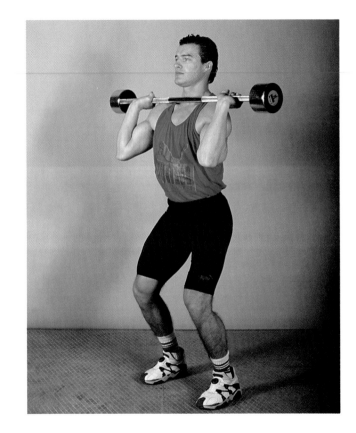

Safety for pupils and competitors

Weight training, i.e. strength and muscle building, is a very worthwhile end in itself. It assists in the development of skill acquisition and is an important aspect of any physical fitness programme. The sport of weightlifting is exciting, requiring great speed, strength, mental control, fitness, courage and mastery of technique. Many top athletes employ progressive resistance principles in their training.

The use of weights, however, requires careful thought. The skills of the activity must be learned very thoroughly. Poor technique, reckless advancement of poundages and irresponsible behaviour can cause accidents. Pupils should listen to their coach or teacher and should apply the correct training principles, while coaches should respect the limitations of each individual. Everything should be clear before training is started.

An injury may result from somebody else not thinking, but if you think and behave responsibly you will never hurt yourself or anybody else. *Consider the following.*

● Confidence should not be confused with recklessness; the former is built on knowledge, the latter on ignorance.

● Although weight training and weightlifting are great fun, because you can see and take pride in the progress you are making, to become an expert still takes time – time spent on understanding and mastering each step before moving on to the next. *Don't try to run before you can walk.*

● Before trying the next exercise or training plans and schedules, get and follow advice from your teacher or coach. *The teacher's or coach's job is to ensure that all the experiences you will have from the use of weights will be pleasant ones.*

● *Never train alone*: always have one stand-in at each end of the bar. *The stand-ins should know what you are going to do and when.*

● Keep to your schedule of exercises. Do not advance to poundages without your coach's advice. *Do not sacrifice correct body position for poundage.*

● Do not try to keep up with others who may seem to be making more rapid progress than yourself. Train at your own level and within your own capabilities: *you will make progress.*

● Horse play and practical jokes can be very dangerous. *If you are not getting enough fun out of serious weightlifting work, it's a poor programme.* Wear firm training shoes and warm clothing.

● Check all apparatus before use and after each exercise. Check collars. Make sure they are firmly secured. Make sure all bars are evenly loaded. *Concentrate and be safety-conscious.*

● When you begin thinking about competition lifting, you will need to have followed a sound training programme. Technique must be mastered. Strength and power building must be developed steadily. *Your success in competition will depend upon a controlled and progressive approach to training.*

Index